Gallbladder Diet Cookbook

Recipes and Tips for a Healthy Gallbladder and Digestive Wellness

Coan Meza

Copyright © by Coan Meza2023. All rights reserved.

Before this document is duplicated or reproduced in any manner, the publisher's consent must be gained. Therefore, the contents within can neither be stored electronically, transferred, nor kept in a database. Neither in Part nor full can the document be copied, scanned, faxed, or retained without approval from the publisher or creator.

Table of content

Introduction

Welcome to "Gallbladder Diet Cookbook" If you or a loved one have experienced gallbladder issues or simply wish to maintain a healthy gallbladder, you've made a wise choice by picking up this cookbook.

The gallbladder, a small yet crucial organ in our digestive system, plays a vital role in storing and releasing bile to aid in the digestion of fats. Unfortunately, it can become susceptible to various conditions that may require dietary adjustments.

Whether you're dealing with gallstones or inflammation or you're simply seeking to support your gallbladder's health, this cookbook is here to help.

In these pages, you will discover a diverse collection of recipes designed to be both delicious and gentle on your gallbladder. We've carefully crafted this cookbook to provide you with flavorful meals that won't compromise your digestive well-being.

From hearty breakfasts to satisfying dinners, from wholesome snacks to mindful desserts, we've got your dietary needs covered.

This cookbook, however, is more than only a catalog of recipes. Throughout the chapters, you'll also find valuable insights into gallbladder health, tips for managing symptoms, and guidance on creating balanced meal plans.

Our goal is to empower you with the knowledge and recipes you need to make informed choices for a happier, healthier gallbladder.

So, whether you're embarking on a journey to support your gallbladder health or you simply appreciate good food made with care, let "Gallbladder Diet Cookbook" be your trusted companion.

Together, let's savor the flavors of a gallbladder-friendly diet and embrace the path to digestive wellness.

Here's to your health and culinary enjoyment!

Understanding Your Gallbladder

The gallbladder may be small, but its role in our digestive system is significant. It's essential to understand this tiny yet vital organ.

Anatomy of the Gallbladder

The gallbladder is a small, pear-shaped organ located beneath your liver, on the right side of your abdomen.

The major function of the gallbladder is to store bile generated by the liver. Bile is a yellowish-green fluid that plays a crucial role in digesting fats.

The Role of Bile

Bile is released from the gallbladder into the small intestine when you eat a meal, particularly one that contains fats.

Its primary functions include:

Emulsifying Fats: Bile contains bile acids that break down large fat molecules into smaller ones, making them easier for enzymes to digest.

Aiding Absorption: Bile helps your body absorb fat-soluble vitamins (A, D, E, and K) and other nutrients.

Eliminating Waste: Bile also helps eliminate waste products and toxins from your body.

Common Gallbladder Issues

While the gallbladder serves a vital purpose, it can sometimes encounter problems. Some of the common gallbladder issues include:

Gallstones: These are hardened deposits that can form in the gallbladder, blocking the flow of bile and causing pain.

Gallbladder Inflammation: Cholecystitis, or gallbladder inflammation, may be caused by gallstones or other disorders.

Dysfunctional Gallbladder: In some cases, the gallbladder may not function properly, leading to digestive issues.

The Importance of Diet

Your diet plays a crucial role in gallbladder health. By making dietary choices that reduce the risk of gallstones and minimize stress on your gallbladder, you can support its proper functioning and overall well-being.

In the chapters that follow, you'll find a wide variety of recipes and meal ideas that are gentle on the gallbladder yet delicious to the palate.

These recipes are designed to help you navigate your culinary journey while maintaining gallbladder health.

Now that you have a better understanding of your gallbladder and its significance in digestion, let's embark on a delicious and nurturing adventure toward a healthier you.

The Importance of a Gallbladder-Friendly Diet

Maintaining a gallbladder-friendly diet is not only about enjoying delicious meals; it's also about nurturing an essential organ that plays a critical role in your digestive system.

Let's delve into why a gallbladder-friendly diet is of utmost importance.

Preventing Gallstones

One of the primary reasons for adopting a gallbladder-friendly diet is to reduce the risk of gallstones.

Gallstones are small, hard deposits that can form in the gallbladder. They can range in size from tiny grains of sand to larger pebbles, and they can cause significant discomfort.

Gallstones develop when the balance of substances that make up bile, such as cholesterol and bilirubin, is disrupted.

A diet high in certain fats and cholesterol can contribute to the formation of gallstones. By making mindful dietary choices, you can lower your risk of developing these painful obstructions.

Supporting Gallbladder Function

A gallbladder-friendly diet is not just about preventing gallstones; it's also about supporting the overall function of this organ. When your gallbladder is healthy, it stores and releases bile efficiently, aiding in the digestion of fats.

However, a diet high in saturated and trans fats can overload your gallbladder and strain its function.

By choosing foods that are gentle on the gallbladder, you can help it do its job effectively. This includes selecting meals that are lower in unhealthy fats and rich in fiber, which promotes proper digestion.

Reducing Digestive Discomfort

If you've ever experienced gallbladder issues, you're well aware of the discomfort they can cause.

Symptoms such as abdominal pain, bloating, and nausea can be disruptive to your daily life. Adopting a gallbladder-friendly diet can help alleviate these symptoms and promote digestive comfort.

Promoting Overall Wellness

Lastly, a gallbladder-friendly diet isn't just about addressing immediate concerns—it's part of a broader commitment to your overall well-being.

By making choices that support your gallbladder, you're also promoting a healthier lifestyle.

A diet rich in fruits, vegetables, lean proteins, and whole grains is not only good for your gallbladder but also beneficial for your heart, weight management, and long-term health.

In the chapters that follow, you'll discover a wealth of recipes and meal ideas designed to strike a balance between gastronomic pleasure and gallbladder health. Whether you're proactively caring for your gallbladder or navigating gallbladder issues, this cookbook is your culinary guide to a happier and healthier digestive system.

How to Use This Cookbook

Congratulations on embarking on your journey to nourish your gallbladder and embrace a healthier lifestyle.
This cookbook has been carefully crafted to provide you with the tools and recipes you need to support your

gallbladder's well-being while savoring the pleasures of food. Here is how to go about it:

1. Getting Started

Begin by reading the introductory sections, including "Understanding Your Gallbladder" and "The Importance of a Gallbladder-Friendly Diet." This foundational knowledge will help you appreciate the significance of your gallbladder and the role your diet plays in its health.

2. Exploring the Recipes

The heart of this cookbook lies in its recipes, thoughtfully organized into chapters to cover every meal and snack throughout the day.

Each recipe is designed to be gentle on your gallbladder while maximizing flavor and nutritional value.

Feel free to explore and try recipes that pique your interest.

3. Recipe Selection

Recipes should be picked depending on your dietary choices and limits.

Whether you're a vegetarian, prefer gluten-free options, or have specific taste preferences, you'll find a variety of recipes that cater to your needs.

Each recipe includes a list of ingredients, clear instructions, and serving sizes to make meal planning easy.

4. Meal Planning

To make the most of your gallbladder-friendly diet, consider planning your meals.

The "Meal Planning and Portion Control" chapter offers guidance on creating balanced meal plans that support your gallbladder while satisfying your taste buds.

5. Dietary Modifications

If you have specific dietary requirements or need to make adjustments for medical reasons, this cookbook provides flexibility.

Many recipes can be adapted to suit your needs, whether you need to lower fat content or eliminate certain ingredients.

6. Managing Symptoms

If you're dealing with gallbladder issues, refer to the section on "Managing Gallbladder Symptoms" for tips and lifestyle changes that can help alleviate discomfort and promote healing.

7. Exploring Beverages

Don't forget about beverages! The "Beverages for Digestive Health" chapter offers a selection of drinks that can complement your meals while supporting your digestive system.

8. Seeking Medical Advice

While this cookbook provides valuable dietary guidance, it's essential to consult with a healthcare professional for personalized advice if you have specific medical conditions or concerns related to your gallbladder.

9. Enjoy the Journey

Remember that your journey to gallbladder wellness should also be enjoyable.
Experiment with flavors, discover new ingredients and savor each meal.

Eating well should be a pleasure, and this cookbook aims to make that a reality.

We're excited to join you on this gastronomic adventure towards a healthier and happier gallbladder. Let's get started, one delicious and nurturing recipe at a time!

Chapter 1
Gallbladder Diet Basics

In this chapter, we'll lay the foundation for understanding what a gallbladder-friendly diet entails. We'll explore the key elements of this diet and why they matter for your gallbladder's health.

What Is a Gallbladder Diet?

A gallbladder diet is a specialized eating plan designed to promote the health and well-being of your gallbladder, a small but essential organ in your digestive system. This dietary approach is particularly beneficial for individuals who have experienced gallbladder issues, such as gallstones or inflammation, or for those looking to prevent such problems.

Definition and Purpose

At its core, a gallbladder diet focuses on reducing the risk of gallstones, supporting gallbladder function, and minimizing discomfort associated with gallbladder issues.

Here's a closer look at the primary objectives:

1. **Reducing Gallstone Formation:** Gallstones are solid particles that form in the gallbladder, often due to

imbalances in the composition of bile.

A gallbladder diet aims to lower the risk of gallstone development by moderating dietary factors that contribute to their formation.

2. Supporting Gallbladder Function: A healthy gallbladder efficiently stores and releases bile, which aids in the digestion of fats.

A gallbladder-friendly diet promotes proper gallbladder function, ensuring it can perform its digestive role effectively.

3. Minimizing Discomfort: For individuals with existing gallbladder issues, certain foods can trigger pain, bloating, and other uncomfortable symptoms. A gallbladder diet helps alleviate these symptoms by avoiding problematic foods.

Key Principles

To achieve these, a gallbladder diet is guided by several key principles:

1. **Low in Saturated and Trans Fats:** High-fat diets, especially those rich in saturated and trans fats, can overwork the gallbladder and lead to gallstone formation.

A gallbladder diet limits the intake of these fats.

2. High in Fiber: Fiber aids digestion and helps prevent constipation, which can exacerbate gallbladder issues. Including fiber-rich foods in your diet is a cornerstone of gallbladder health.

3. Lean Proteins: Lean sources of protein, such as poultry, fish, and plant-based options, are preferred over fatty meats to reduce the burden on the gallbladder.

4. Fresh Fruits and Vegetables: A diet rich in fresh produce provides essential vitamins, minerals, and antioxidants while being gentle on the gallbladder.

5. Adequate Hydration: Staying well-hydrated supports overall digestion and can help prevent gallstones.

6. Portion Control: Maintaining appropriate portion sizes prevents overloading the digestive system and minimizes stress on the gallbladder.

7. Mindful Eating: Practicing mindful eating techniques, such as eating slowly and savoring each bite, can enhance digestion and reduce discomfort.

Understanding these fundamental principles of a gallbladder diet is the first step toward fostering a healthier relationship between your diet and your digestive system.

Foods to Avoid

When following a gallbladder-friendly diet, it's crucial to be mindful of the foods that can potentially trigger gallbladder issues or exacerbate existing problems.

By avoiding certain foods, you can reduce the risk of gallstone formation and minimize discomfort.

Here's a closer look at the categories of foods to steer clear of:

1. High-Fat Foods

High-fat foods are a primary concern when it comes to gallbladder health.

Excessive fat intake can overwork the gallbladder and increase the likelihood of gallstone formation.

Foods in this category include:

- Fried chicken, including french fries, are examples of fried foods
- Fatty cuts of meat, like beef or pork, with visible fat
- Processed meats like sausages and bacon
- Full-fat dairy products, including whole milk and high-fat cheeses

- Oils with high saturated fat content, such as coconut oil and palm oil

2. Processed and Fried Foods

Processed and fried foods often contain unhealthy fats, additives, and preservatives that can be harsh on the gallbladder.
Limit or avoid these items:

- Commercially prepared fast food
- Frozen meals high in saturated fats
- Packaged snacks like chips and crackers
- Processed baked goods with trans fats

- Deep-fried foods, including doughnuts and fried appetizers

3. High-Cholesterol Foods

Dietary cholesterol can contribute to the development of gallstones, so it's advisable to reduce the intake of high-cholesterol foods:

- Organ meats like liver and kidneys
- Shellfish such as shrimp and lobster
- Egg yolks (egg whites are a healthier option)
- Foods prepared with excessive amounts of butter or lard

4. Spicy and Rich Foods

Spicy and rich foods can be hard to digest, potentially leading to gallbladder discomfort, especially if you have existing gallbladder issues.

Be cautious with dishes that are:
- Spicy, containing hot peppers or excessive spices
- Rich in cream, butter, or heavy sauces
- High in sugar, as excessive sugar intake can contribute to digestive problems

By being vigilant about these categories of foods to avoid, you can reduce the strain on your gallbladder and minimize the chances of experiencing gallbladder-related discomfort.

Remember that dietary adjustments can have a positive impact on your gallbladder's well-being, making it easier to embrace a lifestyle that supports digestive health.

Foods to Include

A gallbladder-friendly diet isn't just about avoiding problematic foods; it's also about embracing a wide variety of nourishing options that support gallbladder health.

By including certain foods in your diet, you can promote proper digestion, reduce the risk of gallstones, and foster overall well-being.

Here are the key categories of foods to include:

1. Lean Proteins

Lean sources of protein should be a cornerstone of your gallbladder-friendly meals. These proteins provide essential nutrients without overburdening your gallbladder with excess fat. Opt for:

- Skinless poultry, such as chicken or turkey
- Lean cuts of meat, including sirloin, tenderloin, or loin chops
- Fish, particularly varieties like salmon, trout, and cod
- Tofu, tempeh, and legumes (beans, lentils, chickpeas)

are examples of plant-based proteins.

2. Fiber-Rich Foods

Fiber is a digestive ally and plays a crucial role in maintaining gallbladder health.

It helps regulate bowel movements, prevents constipation, and may reduce the risk of gallstone formation. Include:

- Fresh fruits like apples, pears, and berries
- Vegetables, especially leafy greens, broccoli, and cauliflower
- Oatmeal, quinoa, brown rice, and whole wheat pasta

are examples of whole grains
- Legumes such as beans, lentils, and peas

3. Fresh Fruits and Vegetables

A plant-rich diet is particularly beneficial for gallbladder health due to the abundance of vitamins, minerals, and antioxidants.

Aim to incorporate a colorful array of fruits and vegetables, which provide essential nutrients and support overall digestion:

- Swiss including, kale and spinach, are examples of leafy greens
- Berries, rich in antioxidants and fiber

- Lemons, including oranges and grapefruits, are examples of citrus fruits
- Cruciferous vegetables like broccoli and Brussels sprouts
- Colorful bell peppers, carrots, and tomatoes

4. Whole Grains

Whole grains are not only a source of fiber but also provide essential carbohydrates for energy.

They contribute to a well-rounded, gallbladder-friendly diet:

- Oatmeal for a fiber-rich breakfast
- Quinoa, a versatile and protein-packed grain

- Whole wheat bread and pasta
- Brown rice as a nutritious side dish

5. Healthy Fats

While it's important to limit saturated and trans fats, your body still needs healthy fats in moderation. Incorporate sources of these beneficial fats into your diet:

- Avocado is a creamy and nutritious addition to salads and sandwiches
- Nuts like almonds, walnuts, and cashews (in controlled portions)

- Seeds such as chia seeds, flaxseeds, and pumpkin seeds
- Olive oil for cooking and dressings (in moderation)

6. Hydration

Proper hydration supports digestion and helps prevent gallstones.

Consume lots of water throughout the day.

You can also enjoy herbal teas and infusions, which contribute to your daily fluid intake.

By embracing these foods in your gallbladder-friendly diet, you'll not only nurture your digestive system but also enjoy a diverse range of flavors and textures.

Chapter 2
Breakfast Delights

Creamy Oatmeal with Berries is a delightful and gallbladder-friendly breakfast option.

Ingredients:
- 1/2 cup old-fashioned rolled oats
- 1 cup water
- 1/2 cup low-fat or skim milk (or dairy-free alternative)
- 1/2 teaspoon vanilla extract
- 1/4 teaspoon ground cinnamon (optional)
- A cup of fresh berries that is raspberries, strawberries and blueberries

- 1 tbsp honey or maple syrup (optional for added sweetness)
- Chopped nuts (e.g., almonds or walnuts) for garnish (optional)

Instructions:

- Cook the Oats:

Boil a cup of water in a saucepan Stir in the rolled oats and reduce the heat to low. Allow the oats to cook for 5 minutes, stirring regularly.

- Add Milk and Flavorings:

Pour in the milk (or dairy-free alternative) and continue to cook over low heat. If using, stir in the vanilla essence and powdered cinnamon.

Continue cooking for another 3-5 minutes or until the oats reach your desired level of creaminess. Stir constantly to avoid sticking or burning.

- Serve and Sweeten:

Transfer the creamy oatmeal to a bowl.

Top with fresh berries of your choice. Berries are an excellent source of antioxidants and add natural sweetness.

If desired, drizzle with honey or maple syrup for extra sweetness. Keep in mind that sweetness is optional and can be adjusted to your taste.

- Garnish:

Optionally, sprinkle chopped nuts like almonds or walnuts on top for added texture and healthy fats.

- Enjoy:

Serve your creamy oatmeal with berries hot and, savor the delicious and nutritious start to your day!

- Tips:

You can add sliced bananas, a dollop of Greek yogurt, or a sprinkle of ground flaxseed for additional nutrition.

Scrambled Eggs with Herbs are a protein-packed and gallbladder-friendly breakfast option.

Ingredients:
- 2 large eggs

- 1 tablespoon low-fat milk (or dairy-free alternative)
- Salt and pepper to taste
- 1 teaspoon olive oil or cooking spray for the pan
- 1 tablespoon chopped fresh herbs (e.g., chives, parsley, dill)
- Optional: 1/4 cup diced bell peppers, onions, or spinach for added flavor and nutrition

Instructions:
- Prepare Your Eggs:

Crack the eggs into a bowl, add the milk, and season with a bit of salt and pepper to taste.

The eggs should be whisked vigorously until the yolks and

whites are fully mixed and reasonably foamy.

- Heat the Pan:

Place a non-stick skillet over medium-low heat and add the olive oil or a spritz of cooking spray.

Sauté Optional Vegetables (If Using):

If you're adding diced bell peppers, onions, or spinach, sauté them in the pan until they're tender and slightly caramelized.

This adds extra flavor and nutrients to your scrambled eggs.

- Scramble the Eggs:

Pour the whisked eggs into the pan.

Let them sit undisturbed for a moment until the edges begin to set.

- Add Herbs:

Sprinkle the chopped fresh herbs evenly over the eggs. The herbs not only add flavor but also provide antioxidants and nutrients.

- Gently Scramble:

Gently whisk the eggs in a figure-eight motion using a spatula.

Be patient and avoid overcooking; the eggs should be soft and slightly runny in places.

- Remove from Heat:

Once the eggs are mostly set but still slightly runny on the surface, remove the pan from the heat.

The remaining heat will keep the eggs thoroughly cooked.

- Serve:

Transfer your scrambled eggs with herbs to a plate.
Garnish with a little extra chopped fresh herbs for a burst of color and flavor.

- Enjoy:

Savor your delicious and creamy scrambled eggs with herbs. They're a protein-packed breakfast that's gentle on your gallbladder and bursting with flavor.

- Tips:

You can add different fresh herbs, such as chives, parsley, dill, or basil, to change the flavor profile.

Banana and Almond Butter Smoothie is a quick and nutritious gallbladder-friendly breakfast option

Ingredients:

- 1 ripe banana
- 1 tablespoon almond butter (unsweetened and without added oils)
- 1/2 cup low-fat or skim milk (or dairy-free alternative like almond milk)
- Optional: 1/2 cup Greek yogurt (for additional creaminess and protein).
- 1/2 teaspoon honey (optional for sweetness)

- You may add ice cubes to obtain colder and thicker consistency (optional)

Instructions:

- Prepare the Banana:

Peel the ripe banana and break it into chunks for easier blending.

- Combine Ingredients:

In a blender, add the banana chunks, almond butter, low-fat milk (or dairy-free alternative), and Greek yogurt (if using).

If you prefer a sweeter smoothie, you can add honey at this stage. Keep in mind that sweetness is optional and can be adjusted to your taste.

- Blend Until Smooth:

Blend all of the ingredients until they are creamy and smooth.

If you want a thicker smoothie, you can add a handful of ice cubes and blend until they're fully incorporated.

- Taste and Adjust:

Taste the smoothie and adjust the sweetness or thickness by adding more honey or ice cubes if needed.

Blend briefly to combine any additional ingredients.

- Serve:

Pour your banana and almond butter smoothie into a glass.

- Enjoy:

Sip and enjoy your delicious and nutritious smoothie as a quick and convenient gallbladder-friendly breakfast option.

- Tips:

To make this smoothie even more nutrient-packed, consider adding a handful of fresh spinach or kale. You won't taste the greens, but you'll benefit from their vitamins and fiber.

Vegetable Omelet is a savory and gallbladder-friendly breakfast option.

Ingredients:

- 2 large eggs
- 1/4 cup diced bell peppers (choose your favorite color)
- 1/4 cup diced onions
- 1/4 cup diced tomatoes
- 1/4 cup chopped spinach or kale (optional)

- Salt and pepper to taste
- 1 teaspoon olive oil or cooking spray for the pan
- 2 tablespoons shredded low-fat cheese (optional for added flavor)
- Fresh herbs (e.g., parsley or chives) for garnish (optional)

Instructions:

- Prepare Your Vegetables:

Dice the bell peppers, onions, and tomatoes.

If you're using spinach or kale, chop it finely.

- Whisk the Eggs:

Crack the eggs into a bowl and whisk them until the yolks and whites are well combined.

Season with a pinch of salt and a dash of pepper.

- Heat the Pan:

Place a non-stick skillet over medium-low heat and add the olive oil or a spritz of cooking spray.

- Sauté the Vegetables:

Add the diced bell peppers and onions to the pan.

Sauté them until they become tender and slightly caramelized, usually within 2-3 minutes.

- Add Tomatoes and Greens (If Using):

Stir in the diced tomatoes and chopped spinach or kale, if you're including them. Sauté briefly until the tomatoes are slightly softened.

- Pour in the Eggs:

Spread the sautéed vegetables evenly in the pan.

Pour the whisked eggs over the vegetables.

Allow them to cook without stirring for a moment, allowing the edges to set.

- Add Optional Cheese:

If you're using cheese, sprinkle it evenly over one-half of the omelet.

- Fold the Omelet:

Once the eggs are mostly set but still slightly runny on the top, carefully fold the omelet in half using a spatula.

- Cook Until Set:

Continue cooking for another minute or so, ensuring the eggs are   fully   cooked   but   not overdone.

- Serve:

Slide your vegetable omelet onto a plate.

Enjoy your homemade omelet

Chapter 3
Appetizing Lunches

Grilled Chicken Salad with Lemon Dressing is a delicious and gallbladder-friendly lunch.

Ingredients:
For the Salad:
- 2 boneless, skinless chicken breasts
- 1 tablespoon olive oil (for grilling)
- 6 cups mixed salad greens (lettuce, spinach, arugula, etc.)
- 1 cup cherry tomatoes, halved
- 1/2 cucumber, sliced

- 1/4 red onion, thinly sliced
- 1/4 cup sliced black olives (optional)
- 1/4 cup crumbled feta cheese (optional)
- Salt and pepper to taste

For the Lemon Dressing:
- 3 tablespoons extra-virgin olive oil
- 2 tablespoons fresh lemon juice
- 1 teaspoon Dijon mustard
- 1 clove garlic, minced
- Salt and pepper to taste
- Fresh basil or parsley leaves for garnish (optional)

Instructions:
- Grill the Chicken:

Preheat your grill to medium-high heat. Season both sides of the chicken with salt and pepper.

To prevent the chicken from sticking to the grill, rub it with olive oil.

Grill the chicken for about 6-8 minutes per side or until it reaches an internal temperature of 165°F (74°C) and is no longer pink in the center.

Remove the chicken from the grill and put aside for a few minutes before slicing it into thin strips.

- Prepare the Lemon Dressing:

In a small bowl, whisk together the extra-virgin olive oil, fresh lemon juice, Dijon mustard, minced garlic, salt, and pepper until well combined.

If required, taste and adjust the spices.

- Assemble the Salad:

In a large salad bowl, combine the mixed salad greens, cherry tomatoes, sliced cucumber, red onion, and black olives (if using). Add the sliced grilled chicken on top.

- Drizzle with Lemon Dressing:

Drizzle the lemon dressing over the salad. Toss everything lightly with the dressing to coat the salad.

- Garnish and Serve:

If desired, sprinkle crumbled feta cheese on top and garnish with fresh basil or parsley leaves.

Serve your grilled chicken salad immediately as a nutritious and satisfying meal.

Tips:

You can add vegetables like bell peppers, carrots, or avocado.

If you prefer a vegetarian version, you can omit the chicken and enjoy the salad with additional protein sources like chickpeas or tofu.

Quinoa and Chickpea Salad is a healthy and gallbladder-friendly dish that's perfect for lunch or dinner

Ingredients:

For the Salad:

- 1 cup quinoa, rinsed and drained
- 2 cups water or vegetable broth (for quinoa boiling)
- Rinsed and drained chickpeas 1 can (15 ounces)
- 1 cup cherry tomatoes, halved
- 1 cucumber, diced
- 1/4 cup red onion, finely chopped
- 1/4 cup fresh parsley, chopped
- 1/4 cup fresh mint leaves, chopped (optional)
- Salt and pepper to taste

For the Dressing:

- 1/4 cup extra-virgin olive oil

- 2 tablespoons fresh lemon juice
- 1 clove garlic, minced
- 1 teaspoon Dijon mustard
- Salt and pepper to taste

Instructions:
- Cook the Quinoa:

In a medium saucepan, combine the rinsed quinoa and water or vegetable broth. Over medium-high heat, bring to a boil.

Reduce the heat to low, cover, and simmer for about 15-20 minutes or until the quinoa is tender and has absorbed the liquid.

Remove from heat and let it cool.
- Prepare the Dressing:

In a small bowl, whisk together the extra-virgin olive oil, fresh lemon juice, minced garlic, Dijon mustard, salt, and pepper until well combined. Add salt and pepper to taste.

- Assemble the Salad:

In a large salad bowl, combine the cooked and cooled quinoa, chickpeas, halved cherry tomatoes, diced cucumber, chopped red onion, fresh parsley, and optional fresh mint leaves. Season with salt and pepper to taste.

- Drizzle with Dressing:

Drizzle the lemon and olive oil dressing over the salad ingredients.

- Toss and Serve:

Gently toss all the ingredients together until the salad is well coated with the dressing.

- Chill and Enjoy:

Refrigerate the quinoa and chickpea salad for at least 30 minutes to allow the flavors to meld.

Serve chilled as a delicious, protein-packed, and gallbladder-friendly meal.

Tips:

You can add vegetables, such as diced bell peppers, grated carrots, or avocado.

Salmon and Avocado Wrap is a delicious and gallbladder-friendly lunch or dinner option.

Ingredients:
- 2 salmon fillets, skinless and boneless
- Salt and pepper to taste
- 1 tablespoon olive oil
- 2 whole-grain or spinach tortillas or wraps
- 1 ripe avocado, sliced
- 1 cup mixed greens (e.g., spinach, arugula, or lettuce)
- 1/4 cup red onion, thinly sliced
- 1/4 cup cucumber, thinly sliced

- 2 tablespoons Greek yogurt or sour cream (optional for added creaminess)
- Lemon wedges for garnish (optional)

Instructions:

- Prepare the Salmon:

Add salt and pepper to taste.

In a skillet over medium-high heat, add the olive oil.

Place the salmon fillets in the skillet and cook for about 3-4 minutes per side or until the salmon is cooked through and flakes easily with a fork.

Remove it from the skillet and allow it to cool for some minutes.

- Assemble the Wraps:

Lay out the tortillas or wraps on a clean surface.

Divide the sliced avocado, mixed greens, red onion, and cucumber evenly between the two wraps, placing the ingredients down the center of each tortilla.

- Flake the Salmon:

Use a fork to flake the cooked salmon into bite-sized pieces.

- Add Salmon to Wraps:

Divide the flaked salmon evenly between the wraps, placing it on top of the other ingredients.

- Optional Creamy Element:

If you'd like to add creaminess to your wraps, drizzle 1 tablespoon of Greek yogurt or sour cream over each wrap.

- Fold and Serve:

Carefully fold the sides of each tortilla over the filling.
Roll up the wraps tightly from the bottom to enclose the ingredients.
You can still slice each wrap in half diagonally if you desire.

- Garnish (Optional):

Garnish with lemon wedges for an extra burst of flavor.

- Enjoy:

Serve your salmon and avocado wraps immediately as a nutritious and satisfying meal.

Tips:

You can customize your wraps by adding other ingredients, such as diced tomatoes, grated carrots, or a sprinkle of fresh herbs like dill or cilantro.

To make these wraps even heartier, you can add a small amount of cooked quinoa or brown rice inside.

Lentil Soup makes a comforting and nutritious meal.

Ingredients:
- Rinsed and drained 1 cup of dried green or brown lentils,
- 1 tablespoon olive oil
- 1 onion, chopped
- 2 carrots, diced
- 2 celery stalks, diced
- 2 cloves garlic, minced
- 1 teaspoon ground cumin
- 1/2 teaspoon ground coriander
- 1/2 teaspoon paprika

- 1/4 teaspoon ground turmeric
- 1 bay leaf
- 6 cups low-sodium vegetable broth or water
- 1 can (14 ounces) diced tomatoes (with juices)
- Salt and pepper to taste
- Fresh lemon juice (optional for serving)
- Fresh parsley or cilantro leaves for garnish (optional)

Instructions:

- Prepare Lentils:

Rinse the lentils under cold running water and drain them.

- Sauté Vegetables:

In a pot, heat the olive oil.

Put together the chopped onion, diced carrots, and diced celery. Allow it for about 5 minutes.

- Add Spices:

Stir in the minced garlic, ground cumin, ground coriander, paprika, ground turmeric, and bay leaf.

You have to cook for about a minute to make the spices more fragrant.

- Combine Lentils and Liquid:

Add the rinsed lentils, vegetable broth (or water), and diced tomatoes (with juices) to the pot. Stir everything together.

- Simmer:

Bring the mixture to a boil, then reduce the heat to low, cover the pot, and let it simmer for about

20-25 minutes or until the lentils and vegetables are tender. Be sure to stir occasionally.

- Season:

Season it with salt and pepper to taste. Adjust the seasoning to your preference.

- Serve:

Ladle the lentil soup into bowls. Optionally, squeeze fresh lemon juice over each serving for a bright and zesty flavor.

Garnish with fresh parsley or cilantro leaves if desired.

- Enjoy:

Serve your homemade lentil soup hot and savor the comforting and nutritious flavors.

Tips:

You can add vegetables like spinach, kale, or diced potatoes. If you prefer a smoother texture, you can use an immersion blender to partially blend the soup, leaving some lentils and vegetables intact.

Chapter 4
Satisfying Dinners

Baked Cod with Garlic and Herbs is a delicious and gallbladder-friendly dinner option.

Ingredients:
- Skinless and boneless
- 4 cod fillets (like 6 ounces each),
- 2 tablespoons olive oil
- 3 cloves garlic, minced
- Dried thyme 1 teaspoon (or fresh thyme leaves 1 tablespoon)
- 1 teaspoon dried rosemary (or 1 tablespoon fresh rosemary leaves, chopped)

- Dried oregano 1 teaspoon (or fresh oregano leaves 1 tablespoon)
- Salt and pepper to taste
- Lemon wedges for serving (optional)
- Fresh parsley or dill leaves for garnish (optional)

Instructions:

- Preheat the Oven:

Preheat your oven to 375°F (190°C).

- Prepare the Herbed Olive Oil:

In a small bowl, combine the olive oil, minced garlic, dried thyme, dried rosemary, and dried oregano.

Mix well to create a flavorful herb-infused olive oil.

- Season the Cod:

With paper towels, pat the cod fillets dry

Add both sides of the cod fillets with salt and pepper to taste.

- Arrange in a Baking Dish:

Place the cod fillets in a baking dish large enough to hold them without crowding.

- Brush with Herbed Olive Oil:

Brush the herbed olive oil mixture evenly over the top of each cod fillet.

- Bake:

Bake the cod in the preheated oven for approximately 12-15 minutes or until the fish is opaque and flakes easily with a fork.

The exact cooking time may vary based on the thickness of the fillets, so keep an eye on them to avoid overcooking.

  • Garnish and Serve:

Once the cod is done, remove it from the oven.

Garnish with fresh parsley or dill leaves if desired.

Optionally, serve with lemon wedges for a zesty touch.

  • Enjoy:

Serve your baked cod with garlic and herbs immediately as a flavorful and gallbladder-friendly dinner.

Turkey and Vegetable Stir-Fry is a tasty and gallbladder-friendly dinner option.

Ingredients:
For the Stir-Fry Sauce:
- Low-sodium soy sauce 2 tablespoons
- 1 tablespoon rice vinegar
- 1 tablespoon honey or maple syrup
- 1 teaspoon cornstarch (or arrowroot powder for a gluten-free option)
- 1/4 cup water

For the Stir-Fry:
- 1 pound lean ground turkey
- 1 tablespoon olive oil
- 1 onion, thinly sliced
- 2 cloves garlic, minced

- 1 bell pepper, thinly sliced (use your favorite color)
- 1 zucchini, thinly sliced
- 1 carrot, thinly sliced
- 1 cup broccoli florets
- Salt and pepper to taste
- Cooked brown rice or quinoa for serving
- Green onions for garnish (optional)

Instructions:

- Prepare the Stir-Fry Sauce:

In a small bowl, whisk together the low-sodium soy sauce, rice vinegar, honey or maple syrup, cornstarch (or arrowroot powder), and water until well combined. Set aside.

- Cook the Ground Turkey:

In a large wok, heat the olive oil on a medium-high heat.

Add the ground turkey and cook, breaking it apart with a spoon, until it's no longer pink and is cooked through.

Bring it down from the skillet and set aside.

- Sauté the Vegetables:

Add a little more olive oil in the same skillet if needed.

Add the thinly sliced onion and minced garlic.

Sauté for about 2 minutes or until the onion becomes translucent and aromatic.

- Add the Remaining Vegetables:

Add the thinly sliced bell pepper, zucchini, carrot, and broccoli florets to the skillet.

Stir-fry the vegetables for approximately 5-7 minutes or until they're tender-crisp.

You want them to maintain their vibrant colors and some crunch.

- Combine with Ground Turkey:

Return the cooked ground turkey to the skillet with the sautéed vegetables. Mix everything.

- Add the Stir-Fry Sauce:

Pour the prepared stir-fry sauce over the turkey and vegetables in the skillet.

- Cook and Thicken:

Cook for another 2-3 minutes to make the sauce thicken and coat the ingredients. Stir occasionally.

- Season and Serve:

Add salt and pepper to taste.

Serve your turkey and vegetable stir-fry hot cooked brown rice or quinoa.

- Garnish and Enjoy:

If desired, garnish with fresh cilantro or chopped green onions for extra flavor and visual appeal.

Tips

You can add vegetables like snap peas, mushrooms, or baby corn.

Adjust the level of heat by adding red pepper flakes or sriracha sauce if you enjoy a bit of spice.

Roasted Vegetable Medley is a delightful and gallbladder-friendly side dish or even a main course if you like.

Ingredients:

- 2 cups mixed vegetables (e.g., carrots, bell peppers, zucchini, cherry tomatoes, broccoli, cauliflower, and red onion), washed, peeled, and chopped into bite-sized pieces
- 2 tablespoons olive oil
- Dried thyme 1 teaspoon (or fresh thyme leaves 1 tablespoon)
- 1 teaspoon dried rosemary (or 1 tablespoon fresh rosemary leaves, chopped)

- Salt and pepper to taste
- Optional: 2 cloves garlic, minced
- Optional: Grated Parmesan cheese for garnish (skip if dairy is a concern)

Instructions:
- Preheat the Oven:

Preheat your oven to 400°F (200°C).
- Prepare the Vegetables:

You have to wash, peel, and chop the mixed vegetables into bite-sized pieces. You can take a variety of vegetables as you prefer.
- Season and Toss:

In a large bowl, combine the chopped vegetables, olive oil,

dried thyme, dried rosemary, salt, and pepper.

You can add minced garlic for extra flavor if you wish.

Toss everything together until the vegetables are evenly coated with olive oil and seasonings.

- Arrange on a Baking Sheet:

On a baking sheet, arrange the seasoned vegetables in a single layer. Make sure they're not crowded to allow for even roasting.

- Roast in the Oven:

Roast the vegetable medley in the preheated oven for approximately 20-25 minutes or until the vegetables are tender and lightly browned.

Stir or toss them halfway through the cooking time for even roasting.

- Serve and Garnish:

Hence, the vegetables are roasted very well and brought down from the oven.

Optionally, garnish with grated Parmesan cheese for added flavor.

- Enjoy:

Serve your roasted vegetable medley as a delicious and gallbladder-friendly side dish, or enjoy it as a main course with a side of quinoa or rice.

Tips:

You can also experiment with different herbs and spices to change up the flavor profile.

Fresh herbs like basil or parsley also work well.

Brown Rice Pilaf is a flavorful and gallbladder-friendly side dish.

Ingredients:
- 1 cup brown rice
- 2 cups low-sodium vegetable broth (or chicken broth if preferred)
- 1 tablespoon olive oil or butter
- 1 small onion, finely chopped
- 2 cloves garlic, minced
- 1/4 cup diced carrots
- 1/4 cup diced celery
- 1/4 cup diced bell peppers (choose your favorite color)

- 1/4 cup frozen peas (thawed)
- 1/4 cup sliced almonds or pine nuts (optional)
- Dried thyme 1 teaspoon (or fresh thyme leaves 1 tablespoon)
- Salt and pepper to taste
- Fresh parsley or chives for garnish (optional)

Instructions:

- Rinse and Drain the Rice:

Under cold running water Rinse the brown rice until the water runs clear. Drain the rice.

- Sauté the Aromatics:

In a saucepan, heat the olive oil or butter on a medium heat.

Add the finely chopped onion and cook for about 2-3 minutes until it becomes translucent and aromatic.

● Add Vegetables and Nuts:
Stir in the minced garlic, diced carrots, diced celery, and diced bell peppers.
Cook for another 3-4 minutes until the vegetables begin to soften.
If you're using sliced almonds or pine nuts, add them to the pan and toast them for about 2-3 minutes until they turn lightly golden.

● Toast the Rice:
Add the rinsed and drained brown rice to the skillet with the sautéed vegetables. Stir and

cook for 2-3 minutes to toast the rice slightly.

- Add Broth and Seasonings:

Pour in the low-sodium vegetable or chicken broth and add the dried thyme. Add salt and pepper to taste.

Boil the mixture, then reduce the heat, cover, and simmer. Cook according to the rice package instructions, usually around 45-50 minutes, or until the rice is tender and has absorbed the liquid.

- Fluff and Garnish:

Hence, the rice is cooked, with a fork fluff it to separate the grains. Optionally, garnish with fresh parsley or chives for added freshness and flavor.

- Serve:

Serve your brown rice pilaf hot as a flavorful and gallbladder-friendly side dish.

Tips:

Customize your brown rice pilaf by adding other vegetables or herbs that you enjoy. Mushrooms, asparagus, or fresh basil can be delicious additions.

Chapter 5
Tasty Snacks and Sides

Greek Yogurt and Cucumber Dip
also known as Tzatziki, is a
fantastic and gallbladder-friendly
dip or condiment.

Ingredients:
- 1 cup Greek yogurt (full-fat or low-fat, depending on your preference)
- 1 cucumber, finely grated
- 2 cloves garlic, minced
- 1 tablespoon extra-virgin olive oil
- 1 tablespoon fresh lemon juice

- Well chopped fresh dill 1 tablespoon (or dried dill 1 teaspoon,)
- Salt and pepper to taste

Instructions:

- Prepare the Cucumber:

Wash and peel the cucumber. Grate it using a fine grater.

- Drain the Cucumber:

Place the grated cucumber in a fine-mesh sieve or a clean kitchen towel.

Sprinkle a little salt over the cucumber and let it sit for about 10-15 minutes. This helps draw out excess moisture from the cucumber.

- Squeeze and Drain:

After letting the cucumber sit, squeeze it tightly in the kitchen towel or sieve to remove as much liquid as possible.

- Mix the Ingredients:

In a mixing bowl, combine the Greek yogurt, minced garlic, extra-virgin olive oil, fresh lemon juice, and finely chopped dill.

Add the drained-grated cucumber to the mixture. Make a thorough mixture of the ingredients.

- Season:

Add the dip with salt and pepper to taste. Remember that the cucumber has already been salted, so taste before adding more salt.

- Chill:

Cover the bowl with plastic wrap and refrigerate the dip for at least 30 minutes before serving. Chilling allows the flavors to meld.

- Serve:

Serve your Greek yogurt and cucumber dip cold as a refreshing and gallbladder-friendly dip or condiment.

- Enjoy:

Enjoy your homemade Tzatziki dip with pita bread, fresh vegetables, grilled meats, or as a topping for gyros or sandwiches.

Baked Sweet Potato Fries are a delicious and gallbladder-friendly alternative to traditional potato fries:

Ingredients:
- 2 large sweet potatoes
- 2 tablespoons olive oil
- 1 teaspoon paprika
- 1/2 teaspoon garlic powder
- 1/2 teaspoon onion powder
- 1/2 teaspoon dried thyme
- Salt and pepper to taste
- Optional: Fresh parsley or cilantro leaves for garnish

Instructions:
- Preheat the Oven:

Make the oven ready by preheating it to 425°F (220°C)

and, with parchment paper or a silicone baking mat, line a baking sheet.

- Prepare the Sweet Potatoes:

Wash and peel the sweet potatoes.

Cut the sweet potatoes into even-sized fries or wedges. Let them be in uniform thickness to ensure even cooking.

- Season the Fries:

In a large bowl, toss the sweet potato fries with olive oil, paprika, garlic powder, onion powder, dried thyme, salt, and pepper. Make sure the fries are evenly coated with the seasoning.

- Arrange on the Baking Sheet:

Spread the seasoned sweet potato fries in a single layer on the prepared baking sheet, ensuring they are not crowded. Crowding the fries can lead to uneven cooking and less crispiness.

- Bake:

Bake in the preheated oven for about 20-30 minutes, flipping the fries halfway through the cooking time to ensure they brown evenly.

- Check for Doneness:

The fries are done when they are tender on the inside and crispy on the outside. Cooking times may vary based on the thickness of your fries, so keep an eye on them.

- Garnish and Serve:

Once the sweet potato fries are done, remove them from the oven.

Optionally, garnish with fresh parsley or cilantro leaves for added freshness and flavor.

- Enjoy:

Serve your baked sweet potato fries hot as a flavorful and gallbladder-friendly side dish or snack.

Guacamole and Whole Wheat Chips

are a delicious and gallbladder-friendly snack or appetizer:

Ingredients:

For the Guacamole:

- 3 ripe avocados

- 1 small red onion, finely chopped
- 2 cloves garlic, minced
- 1-2 ripe tomatoes, diced
- Juice of 1-2 limes (adjust to taste)
- 1/4 cup fresh cilantro, chopped
- Salt and pepper to taste
- Optional: Jalapeño pepper, finely chopped (for added heat)

For the Whole Wheat Chips:
- Whole wheat tortillas
- Olive oil or cooking spray
- Salt to taste
- Optional: Paprika or chili powder for added flavor

Instructions:

- Prepare the Guacamole:

You will start by cutting the avocados in half, remove the pits, and scoop the flesh into a clean bowl.

Mash the avocado with a fork to your desired level of chunkiness.

Add the finely chopped red onion, minced garlic, diced tomatoes, lime juice, and chopped cilantro to the mashed avocado.

If you like a bit of heat, you can add finely chopped jalapeño pepper at this stage.

Add salt and pepper to taste in the guacamole.

Mix everything until well combined.

- Make Whole Wheat Chips:

Preheat your oven to 350°F (175°C).

Lightly brush or spray both sides of whole wheat tortillas with olive oil or cooking spray. Alternatively, you can use a silicone brush to apply a thin layer of olive oil.

Cut the tortillas into wedges or triangles using a sharp knife or kitchen scissors.

In a single layer, arrange the tortilla wedges on a baking sheet.

Sprinkle with salt and, if desired, paprika or chili powder for added flavor.

- Bake the Whole Wheat Chips:

Place the baking sheet in the preheated oven and bake for

about 10-15 minutes or until the chips are golden brown and crispy. Make a frequent check on them to avoid burning.

- Serve:

Remove the chips from the oven and let them cool slightly.

Serve the freshly baked whole wheat chips with the homemade guacamole.

- Enjoy:

Dip the chips into the guacamole and savor this delightful and gallbladder-friendly snack or appetizer.

Fresh Fruit Salad

Ingredients:

- 2 cups of mixed fresh fruits (such as strawberries, blueberries, grapes, kiwi, pineapple, melon, and oranges), washed, peeled, and diced
- 1 tablespoon honey (optional for added sweetness)
- 1 tablespoon fresh lime or lemon juice
- Fresh mint leaves for garnish (optional)

Instructions:
- Prepare the Fruits:

Wash, peel, and dice the mixed fresh fruits of your choice. You can use any combination that you prefer or what's in season.

- Combine the Fruits:

In a large mixing bowl, combine the diced fruits. You can choose a variety of colors and textures to make the salad visually appealing.

- Add Sweetener and Citrus Juice:

If you desire extra sweetness, drizzle honey over the mixed fruits.

Squeeze fresh lime or lemon juice over the fruits to enhance their flavors and keep them from browning.

- Gently Toss:

Gently toss the fruits to ensure they are coated with the honey and citrus juice.

- Chill:

Cover the fruit salad with plastic wrap or a lid and refrigerate for at least 30 minutes before serving. Chilling allows the flavors to meld and the salad to become refreshingly cold.

- Garnish:

If desired, garnish with fresh mint leaves for added fragrance and presentation.

- Serve:

Serve your fresh fruit salad chilled as a healthy and gallbladder-friendly dessert, snack, or side dish.

Chapter 6
Desserts with Care

Baked Apples with Cinnamon are a warm and comforting dessert or snack.

Ingredients:
- medium-sized apples 4 pieces(Honeycrisp or Granny Smith)
- 2 tablespoons unsalted butter (or coconut oil for a dairy-free option)
- 2 tablespoons honey or maple syrup
- 1 teaspoon ground cinnamon

- 1/4 teaspoon ground nutmeg (optional)
- 1/4 cup chopped nuts (such as walnuts or pecans, optional)
- Ice cream or Vanilla yogurt for serving (optional)

Instructions:

- Preheat the Oven:

Preheat your oven to 350°F (175°C).

- Core the Apples:

Wash the apples and remove the cores using an apple core or a small knife, leaving the bottom intact to create a well for the filling.

- Prepare the Filling:

In a small saucepan, melt the coconut oil or unsalted butter over low heat.

Stir in the honey (or maple syrup), ground cinnamon, and ground nutmeg if using. Mix until the ingredients are well combined and create a fragrant sauce.

- Fill the Apples:

Place the cored apples in a baking dish.

Carefully spoon the cinnamon and honey mixture into each apple, distributing it evenly among them.

- Optional Nuts:

If you'd like to add some crunch and flavor, you can sprinkle chopped nuts over the top of each apple.

- Bake:

Cover the baking dish with aluminum foil.

Bake the apples in the preheated oven for about 30-40 minutes or until the apples are tender. Baking time may vary depending on the size and variety of the apples.

- Check for Doneness:

To check if the apples are done, insert a fork or knife into one of them. It should glide in easily when the apples are tender.

- Serve:

Remove the baked apples from the oven.

Optionally, serve them warm with a scoop of vanilla yogurt or ice cream for added richness.

- Enjoy:

Enjoy your baked apples with cinnamon as a comforting and gallbladder-friendly dessert or snack.

Berry Parfait is a delightful dessert or breakfast option.

Ingredients:
- 1 cup plain Greek yogurt (full-fat or low-fat, depending on your preference)
- 2 cups mixed berries (such as strawberries, blueberries, raspberries, and

blackberries), washed and hulled if needed
- Maple syrup or honey 2 tablespoons (add to taste)
- 1/2 cup granola (look for a low-fat and low-sugar option if desired)
- Fresh mint leaves for garnish (optional)

Instructions:

- Prepare the Berries:

Wash and prepare the mixed berries by removing any stems or hulls. You can use a single type of berry or a combination of your favorites.

- Sweeten the Yogurt:

In a bowl, mix the plain Greek yogurt with honey or maple

syrup, adjusting the sweetness to
your taste.

- Layer the Parfait:

Use clear glasses or parfait
dishes for a visually appealing
presentation.
Begin by adding a spoonful of
sweetened Greek yogurt to the
bottom of each glass.

- Add Berries:

Layer a portion of mixed berries
on top of the yogurt.

- Continue Layering:

Repeat the layering process,
adding another spoonful of
yogurt followed by more berries.
Continue until the glass is nearly
full, ending with a final dollop of
yogurt on top.

- Top with Granola:

Sprinkle a generous amount of granola over the yogurt layer in each glass. The granola adds a delightful crunch to the parfait.

- Garnish:

Optionally, garnish with fresh mint leaves for a touch of color and fragrance.

- Serve:

Serve your berry parfait immediately as a delightful and gallbladder-friendly dessert or breakfast option.

Chia Seed Pudding is a nutritious and versatile dish that can be enjoyed for breakfast or as a healthy dessert

Ingredients:

- 1/4 cup chia seeds

- 1 cup unsweetened almond milk (or your choice of milk, such as coconut milk, soy milk, or cow's milk)
- Honey or maple syrup 1-2 tablespoons (adjust to taste)
- 1/2 teaspoon vanilla extract
- Fresh berries, sliced bananas, or other fruit for topping (optional)
- Chopped nuts or seeds for garnish (optional)

Instructions:

- Combine Chia Seeds and Liquid:

In a bowl, combine the chia seeds and unsweetened almond milk (or your chosen milk). Stir well to evenly distribute the seeds in the liquid.

- Add Sweetener and Flavor:

Mix in the honey or maple syrup for sweetness and the vanilla extract for flavor. Adjust the sweetness to your liking.

- Stir and Rest:

Stir the mixture thoroughly, making sure the chia seeds are well incorporated. You'll notice that the seeds start to absorb the liquid.

- Refrigerate:

Transfer the mixture to an airtight container, or you can cover the bowl with plastic wrap.

Refrigerate the chia seed pudding for at least 2-3 hours or overnight.

The chia seeds will absorb the liquid and thicken during this time, producing a pudding-like texture.

- Stir Again:

After the resting period, give the pudding a good stir to break up any clumps and ensure a smooth texture.

- Serve:

Divide the chia seed pudding into serving bowls or glasses.

- Add Toppings:

Top your chia seed pudding with fresh berries, sliced bananas, or your choice of fruit.

Optionally, garnish with chopped nuts or seeds for added texture and nutrition.

- Enjoy:

Enjoy your gallbladder-friendly chia seed pudding as a satisfying and healthy breakfast or dessert.

Dark Chocolate Avocado Mousse is a creamy and indulgent dessert.

Ingredients:
- 2 ripe avocados, peeled and pitted
- 1/4 cup unsweetened cocoa powder
- Honey or maple syrup ¼ cup (adjust to taste)
- 1/4 cup almond milk (or your choice of milk)
- 1 teaspoon vanilla extract
- A pinch of salt
- Optional toppings: fresh berries, sliced bananas,

chopped nuts, or shaved dark chocolate

Instructions:

- Blend the Avocado:

In a food processor, add the ripe avocados, unsweetened cocoa powder, almond milk, honey or maple syrup, vanilla extract, and a pinch of salt.

- Blend Until Smooth:

Blend the ingredients until it becomes smooth and creamy. You may need to scrape down the sides of the blender or food processor and blend again to ensure everything is well combined.

- Taste and Adjust:

Taste the mousse and adjust the sweetness to your liking by adding more honey or maple syrup if necessary.

- Chill:

Transfer the dark chocolate avocado mousse to serving dishes or small bowls.

- Refrigerate:

Cover the dishes with plastic wrap or lids and refrigerate for at least 30 minutes to allow the mousse to chill and set.

- Serve:

Before serving, you can garnish the mousse with fresh berries, sliced bananas, chopped nuts, or shaved dark chocolate.

- Enjoy:

Enjoy your gallbladder-friendly dark chocolate avocado mousse as a rich and satisfying dessert.

Chapter 7
Beverages for Digestive Health

Ginger tea is known for its digestive benefits and calming properties.

Ingredients:
- 1 to 2 inches of fresh ginger root, peeled and thinly sliced (adjust to taste)
- 2 cups of water
- Honey or lemon slices (optional for added flavor)

Instructions:
- Prepare the Ginger:

Peel the ginger root and slice it into thin rounds or strips. You can adjust the amount of ginger to your preferred level of spiciness.

- Boil the Water:

In a saucepan, boil 2 cups of water.

- Add Ginger:

Once the water is boiling, add the thinly sliced ginger to the pot.

- Simmer:

Reduce the heat to low, cover the saucepan, and let the ginger simmer in the hot water for about 10-15 minutes. This allows the ginger to infuse its flavor into the water.

- Strain:

After simmering, strain the ginger tea into your cup or mug, removing the ginger slices.

- Sweeten (Optional):

If desired, you can sweeten your ginger tea with honey. Adjust the sweetness to your taste.

- Add Lemon (Optional):

For an extra zesty flavor, you can add a slice of lemon to your ginger tea.

- Enjoy:

Sip and savor your gallbladder-friendly ginger tea as a calming beverage.

Tips:

You can enjoy it hot or cold, depending on your choice and the weather.

To store any leftover ginger tea, refrigerate it and reheat it when you're ready to enjoy it again.

Cucumber and Mint Infused Water is a hydrating and flavorful beverage.

Ingredients:

- 1 cucumber, washed and thinly sliced
- A handful of fresh mint leaves, washed
- 2 quarts (8 cups) of filtered water
- Ice cubes (optional)
- Slices of lemon or lime (optional for added zing)

Instructions:

- Prepare the Ingredients:

Wash the cucumber and slice it thinly. You can leave the skin on for added flavor and nutrients. Wash the fresh mint leaves.

- Combine Cucumber and Mint:

In a large pitcher, add fresh mint leaves and the sliced cucumber.

- Add Water:

Pour the filtered water over the cucumber and mint in the pitcher.

- Refrigerate:

Place it in the refrigerator to chill after covering the pitcher. Allow the flavors to infuse for at least 1-2 hours or overnight for a more intense flavor.

- Serve:

When ready to serve, you can add ice cubes to individual glasses for an extra refreshing touch.

Optionally, garnish with slices of lemon or lime for a zesty twist.

- Enjoy:

Sip and enjoy your gallbladder-friendly cucumber and mint-infused water as a revitalizing and hydrating beverage.

Green Smoothie packed with leafy greens and fruits.

Ingredients:

- 2 cups fresh spinach or kale leaves, washed and stems removed

- 1 ripe banana
- 1/2 cup fresh or frozen pineapple chunks
- 1/2 cup fresh or frozen mango chunks
- 1/2 cup plain Greek yogurt (full-fat or low-fat, depending on your preference)
- Unsweetened almond milk 1 cup (or any choice of milk)
- Honey or maple syrup 1 tablespoon (adjust to taste)
- 1/2 teaspoon fresh ginger, grated (optional for added flavor)
- Ice cubes (optional for a colder smoothie)

Instructions:

- Prepare the Ingredients:

Wash and remove the stems from the spinach or kale leaves.

Peel the ripe banana and break it into chunks.

Measure out the pineapple and mango chunks, yogurt, almond milk, honey or maple syrup, and grated ginger (if using).

- Blend the Greens:

Start by blending the spinach or kale leaves with the almond milk until they are well incorporated and smooth. This ensures a smoother texture in your smoothie.

- Add the Fruits and Yogurt:

Add the ripe banana, pineapple chunks, mango chunks, plain Greek yogurt, and grated ginger (if using) to the blender.

- Sweeten and Blend:

Add the honey or maple syrup for sweetness.

If you prefer a colder smoothie, you can add a few ice cubes as well.

Blend all the ingredients until you achieve a creamy and smooth consistency.

- Adjust consistency:

If your smoothie is too thick, you can add more almond milk to reach your desired texture.

- Serve:

Pour your gallbladder-friendly green smoothie into a glass.

- Enjoy:

Sip and enjoy your nutritious green smoothie as a wholesome

and refreshing breakfast or snack.

Herbal Tea Blends

Creating your herbal tea blends can be a delightful and personalized way to enjoy a variety of flavors while tailoring your teas to suit your preferences and specific needs. Here are some popular herbs and ingredients you can use to create your herbal tea blends:

1. Chamomile:

Camomile is an excellent base for soothing herbal teas.

2. Peppermint:

Peppermint leaves add a refreshing and invigorating flavor to teas.

Combines well with other herbs like chamomile or lemon balm.

3. Lavender:

Lavender imparts a fragrant and relaxing quality to teas.

Great for blending with chamomile or lemon verbena.

4. Lemon Balm:

Lemon balm offers a citrusy and slightly sweet taste.

Combines well with mint or lavender for a soothing tea.

5. Hibiscus Flowers:

Hibiscus flowers provide a tart and vibrant red color.

Great for blending with fruits like berries or citrus peels.

6. Ginger:

Fresh or dried ginger root adds warmth and a spicy kick to teas. Often combined with lemon and honey for a soothing tea.

7. Cinnamon:

Cinnamon sticks or chips add a warm and sweet flavor to teas. Pairs well with cloves and cardamom for a spicy chai blend.

8. Licorice Root:

Licorice root offers a sweet and soothing element to teas. Often used in combination with herbs like marshmallow root or slippery elm.

9. Echinacea:

Echinacea is known for its potential immune-boosting properties.

Blends well with herbs like elderberry and ginger.

10. Lemon Verbena:

Lemon verbena leaves provide a strong lemony flavor and aroma. Complements other citrusy herbs like lemongrass.

11. Elderflower:

Elderflower blossoms add a delicate and floral aroma to teas. Often used in blends with mint or chamomile.

12. Rose Hips:

Rose hips are high in vitamin C and add a subtle tartness to teas. Great for blending with hibiscus or other fruits.

13. Fennel Seeds:

Fennel seeds offer a mild licorice-like flavor.

Pairs well with chamomile or ginger for digestive teas.

14. Cardamom Pods:

Cardamom pods impart a unique spicy and citrusy flavor.

Often used in chai blends with cinnamon and cloves.

15. Nettle Leaves:

Nettle leaves are rich in nutrients and have an earthy, grassy taste.

Blends well with mint or lemon balm for a refreshing tea.

Creating Your Herbal Tea Blend:

- Choose your base herb or herbs.
- Add complementary herbs, spices, or flowers to create a balanced flavor profile.

- Experiment with quantities to find the right balance for your taste.
- Combine the ingredients in a jar and store them in a cool, dark place.
- To make tea, use 1-2 teaspoons of the herbal blend per cup of hot water. Allow to steep for 5-10 minutes or as desired.

Remember to explore and adjust ingredients to create herbal tea blends that cater to your preferences and wellness goals. Whether it's a calming bedtime blend or an invigorating morning mix, homemade herbal teas offer endless possibilities for enjoyment and well-being.

Chapter 8
Meal Planning and Portion Control

Creating a Gallbladder-Friendly Meal Plan

Creating a gallbladder-friendly meal plan involves selecting foods that are easy on the digestive system and low in fat to prevent gallbladder discomfort. Here's a sample meal plan with guidelines on suitable foods and cooking methods:

Breakfast:

Option 1: Oatmeal with Berries and Almond Butter

- 1/2 cup of old-fashioned oats made with water or lactose-free milk
- Fresh or frozen berries (e.g., blueberries, strawberries)
- Almond butter 1 tablespoon (or other nut butter)
- A sprinkle of ground flaxseed for added fiber

Option 2: Scrambled Eggs with Vegetables

- Scrambled eggs made with egg whites or whole eggs (if tolerated)
- Sautéed spinach, bell peppers, and tomatoes in a small amount of olive oil

- A slice of whole-grain toast (optional)

Lunch:

Option 1: Grilled Chicken Salad

- Grilled chicken breast or lean turkey slices
- Mixed greens with cucumber, cherry tomatoes, and bell peppers
- Balsamic vinaigrette dressing (use sparingly)
- A small serving of brown rice or quinoa

Option 2: Lentil Soup

- Homemade or low-sodium store-bought lentil soup
- A side salad with mixed greens, lemon juice, and a drizzle of olive oil

- Whole-grain crackers (choose low-fat options)

Snack:
- A piece of fresh fruit (e.g., apple, pear, or banana)
- 1 small handful of unsalted nuts (almonds or walnuts)

Dinner:

Option 1: Baked Salmon with Steamed Vegetables
- Baked salmon filet seasoned with herbs and lemon
- Steamed broccoli and carrots
- Quinoa or brown rice as a side

Option 2: Turkey and Vegetable Stir-Fry

- Lean ground turkey or turkey breast strips
- Stir-fried vegetables (e.g., bell peppers, zucchini, and broccoli) with minimal oil
- Homemade stir-fry sauce or low-sodium soy sauce
- Serve over brown rice or cauliflower rice

Snack/Dessert:
- Greek yogurt with fresh berries and a drizzle of honey (optional)
- Dark chocolate square (70% cocoa or higher)

Fluids:
- Drink plenty of water throughout the day.

- Herbal teas like ginger, chamomile, or peppermint can be soothing.

Guidelines:

- Limit High-Fat Foods: Avoid or minimize high-fat foods such as fried foods, fatty meats, full-fat dairy, and rich sauces.
- Choose Lean Proteins: Opt for lean protein sources like skinless poultry, fish, lean cuts of meat, and plant-based proteins.
- Healthy Fats: Incorporate healthy fats like olive oil, avocado, and nuts in moderation.
- Fiber-Rich Foods: Include plenty of fiber from whole

grains, fruits, and vegetables to support digestion.

- Portion Control: Watch portion sizes to avoid overeating, which can strain your gallbladder.
- Cooking Methods: Favor baking, grilling, steaming, or sautéing with minimal oil over frying.
- Stay Hydrated: Drinking enough water is essential for overall health and digestion.
- Limit Spices: While some spices like ginger can be soothing, avoid excessive use of spicy or heavily seasoned foods.

Remember that gallbladder issues can vary from person to person, so it's crucial to consult with a healthcare professional or registered dietitian for personalized guidance and adjustments to your meal plan based on your specific needs and tolerances.

Portion control is a key aspect of maintaining a balanced diet and managing your calorie intake. Here are some tips to help you control your portions effectively:

Use Smaller Plates and Bowls: Serve your meals on smaller plates and use smaller bowls. This can trick your brain into thinking you're eating a larger portion than you are.

Divide Your Plate: Use the "plate method" to divide it into sections.

Fill half your plate with vegetables, one-quarter with lean protein, and one-quarter with whole grains or starches.

Practice Mindful Eating: Pay attention to what you're eating and savor each bite.

While eating, avoid distractions like TV or smartphones, as they can lead to overeating.

Pre-Portion Snacks: Instead of eating snacks directly from the bag or container, portion them into small containers or zip-lock bags to avoid overeating.

Read Food Labels: Check serving sizes on food labels to understand how much a single serving contains.

Be mindful of multiple servings in a single package.

Use Measuring Cups and Spoons: When cooking or serving, use measuring cups and spoons to ensure accurate portion sizes.

Share Meals: When dining out, consider sharing an entree with a friend or ordering a half portion if available.

Restaurant portions are often larger than necessary.

Plan Your Snacks: Instead of grazing throughout the day, plan your snacks and portion them in advance.

This can help prevent mindless munching.

Pack Leftovers Quickly: After a meal, immediately portion and store leftovers in containers to avoid going back for seconds.

Practice the Two-Bite Rule: If you want to taste a high-calorie or indulgent treat, take two small bites to satisfy your craving without overindulging.

Listen to Your Hunger Cues: Always listen to your body's hunger and fullness signals. Eat when you're hungry and stop when you're satisfied, not overly full.

Slow Down: Eating too quickly can lead to overeating because your body doesn't have time to signal fullness.

Make sure you chew your food thoroughly and savor each bite.

Use Your Hand as a Guide: Your hand can serve as a handy portion control tool.

For example, a serving of meat should be about the size of your palm, and a serving of nuts should fit in the palm of your hand.

Plan Ahead: Plan your meals and snacks and portion them out accordingly.

This can help you avoid compulsive eating.

Stay Hydrated: Drink a glass of water before meals to help control your appetite.

Hunger for water can be mistaken for hunger for food sometimes.

Practice Portion Control at Buffets: If you're at a buffet, start with a small plate and fill it with mostly vegetables and lean proteins.

Avoid piling on high-calorie options.

Use Apps and Food Scales: There are smartphone apps and kitchen scales that can help you track portion sizes and calorie counts.

Remember that portion control is not about depriving yourself but

about making informed choices
and enjoying food in moderation.

Dining Out with Gallbladder Health in Mind

Dining out while prioritizing gallbladder health can be manageable with some strategic choices and awareness.

Here are some tips for dining out with gallbladder health in mind:

1. Research the Menu in Advance:

Many restaurants now post their menus online.

Take advantage of this to review the menu and identify gallbladder-friendly options before you go.

2. Choose Grilled or Baked Over Fried:

Opt for dishes that are baked or grilled rather than fried.

It reduces the amount of unhealthy fats in your dishes.

3. Ask About Preparation Methods:

Don't hesitate to ask your server how dishes are prepared. Request that your food be prepared with minimal oil or butter.

4. Customize Your Order:

Be willing to customize your order to make it gallbladder-friendly.

Ask for dressings, sauces, or gravies on the side so you can control the amount you use.

5. Go for Lean Proteins:

Choose lean protein sources like turkey, grilled chicken, and fish. Avoid heavily marinated or breaded options.

6. Load Up on Vegetables:

Make vegetables a significant part of your meal.

They are typically low in fat and high in fiber, which is good for your digestive system.

7. Be Mindful of Portion Sizes:

Be conscious of portion sizes, and consider sharing a meal or taking leftovers home if the portions are large.

8. Avoid High-Fat Dressings and Condiments:

Skip creamy dressings and sauces, which are often high in

fat. Opt for vinaigrettes, salsa, or lemon juice instead.

9. Limit Alcohol Consumption:

Excessive alcohol intake can aggravate gallbladder issues. Limit alcohol consumption or choose non-alcoholic options.

10. Stay Hydrated:

Drink plenty of water with your meal to aid digestion and help flush out toxins.

11. Be Cautious with Spicy Foods:

Spicy foods can trigger gallbladder discomfort in some people. If you enjoy spicy cuisine, opt for milder options.

12. Slow Down and Chew Thoroughly:

Eating slowly and chewing your food can help reduce the risk of overeating and digestive discomfort.

13. Consider Special Dietary Requests:

If you have specific dietary restrictions or concerns, don't hesitate to inform your server. Many restaurants can accommodate special requests.

14. Skip Desserts or Choose Wisely:

Desserts are often high in sugar and fats. If you must have dessert, consider options like fresh fruit or sorbet.

15. Take Digestive Enzymes (if advised):

If your healthcare provider recommends them, take digestive enzyme supplements before your meal to assist with digestion.

16. Listen to Your Body:

Listen to how different foods react to your body. If certain dishes consistently trigger discomfort, avoid them.

Remember that everyone's tolerance for certain foods may vary, so it's essential to monitor your body's reactions and make choices that align with your specific gallbladder health needs.

Chapter 9
Managing Gallbladder Symptoms

Recognizing and addressing gallbladder issues is essential for maintaining your digestive health. Here are some common signs and steps to take if you suspect you have gallbladder problems.

Common Signs of Gallbladder Issues:

Abdominal Pain: The most common symptom of gallbladder problems is pain in the upper right or center of the abdomen, which may be sharp or cramp-like.

It can also radiate to the back or right shoulder blade.

Nausea and Vomiting: Gallbladder issues can cause nausea and, in some cases, vomiting.

Indigestion and Bloating: You may experience indigestion, bloating, and discomfort after eating, especially high-fat or greasy meals.

Changes in Stool: Gallbladder problems can lead to changes in stool color, particularly pale or clay-colored stools.

Frequent Heartburn: Some individuals with gallbladder

issues may experience frequent heartburn or acid reflux.

Gas and Belching: Excessive gas and belching can be related to gallbladder problems.

Sudden Intolerance to Fatty Foods: If you suddenly find it difficult to tolerate fatty or fried foods, it could be a sign of gallbladder dysfunction.

Steps to Address Gallbladder Issues:

Consult a Healthcare Professional:

Consult a healthcare provider If you experience persistent or severe symptoms.

They can perform tests, including blood work, ultrasound, or a

HIDA scan, to diagnose gallbladder issues.

Change Your Diet:

In many cases, dietary modifications can help alleviate gallbladder symptoms.

A healthcare provider or registered dietitian can help you create a gallbladder-friendly diet plan. This typically includes:

- Reducing saturated fats and cholesterol.
- Increasing fiber intake.
- Eating smaller, more frequent meals.
- Avoiding or limiting fried, greasy, and high-fat foods.
- Incorporating foods that support gallbladder health, such as fruits, vegetables,

whole grains, and lean proteins.

Medications: Your healthcare provider may prescribe medications to manage gallbladder-related symptoms or to dissolve certain types of gallstones.

Lifestyle Changes: Maintaining a healthy weight and engaging in regular physical activity can help manage gallbladder issues. Avoid crash diets or rapid weight loss, as they can increase the risk of gallstones.

Surgery: In cases of severe gallbladder disease or recurrent gallstone problems, surgery to remove the gallbladder (cholecystectomy) may be recommended.

This process is typically minimally invasive and well-tolerated.

Follow Medical Advice: If surgery or medical treatment is recommended, follow your healthcare provider's advice closely.

Discuss any concerns or questions you have about the procedure or medications.

It's important to address gallbladder issues promptly to prevent complications and improve your overall quality of life.

Always seek guidance from a healthcare provider or specialist for an accurate diagnosis and personalized treatment plan based on your specific condition.

Lifestyle Changes for Gallbladder Health

Making lifestyle changes to support gallbladder health can help prevent gallbladder problems and manage existing conditions.

Here are some lifestyle adjustments that can contribute to gallbladder health:

Maintain a Healthy Weight: Excess body weight, especially obesity, is a risk factor for gallstones.

Aim to achieve and maintain a healthy weight through a balanced diet and regular physical activity.

Eat a Gallbladder-Friendly Diet:

Focus on a diet that is low in saturated and trans fats, as well as cholesterol.

Include plenty of vegetables, whole grains, fruits, and lean protein sources in your meals.

Gradually reduce or eliminate high-fat and fried foods, as well as sugary, processed snacks.

Portion Control:

Be mindful of portion sizes to prevent overeating, which can lead to gallbladder discomfort.

Stay Hydrated:

Drinking an adequate amount of water can help prevent gallstone formation. Focus on at least 8 glasses of water a day.

Fiber Intake:

Include fiber-rich foods in your diet to support digestion and regular bowel movements.

This can help prevent gallstone formation.

Good sources of fiber include legumes, fruits, whole grains, and vegetables.

Regular Physical Activity:

Engage in regular exercise to help maintain a healthy weight and promote overall digestive health. Focus on at least 150 minutes of moderate-intensity exercise each week.

Avoid Rapid Weight Loss:
Avoid crash diets or rapid weight loss programs, as they can increase the risk of gallstone formation.

Limit Alcohol Intake:
Moderate alcohol consumption is generally considered safe for gallbladder health, but excessive alcohol intake should be avoided.

Stop Smoking:
If you smoke, quitting is not only beneficial for your overall health but may also lower your risk of gallbladder problems.

Manage Chronic Conditions:
If you have conditions like diabetes or high cholesterol, work with your healthcare provider to manage them

effectively, as they can increase the risk of gallstone formation.

Stress Management:

Chronic stress can impact digestive health. Incorporate stress-reduction techniques such as mindfulness, meditation, yoga, or deep breathing exercises into your routine.

Medication Review:

Some medications can increase the risk of gallstones.

Consult with your healthcare provider to review your medications if you have concerns.

Gradual Weight Loss:

If you need to lose weight, do so gradually and with a balanced diet. A high level of weight loss can increase the risk of gallstone formation.

Consult a Healthcare Provider:

If you have a family history of gallbladder problems or are experiencing symptoms, consult a healthcare provider for proper evaluation and guidance.

Follow Medical Advice:

If you have a diagnosed gallbladder condition, such as gallstones or gallbladder inflammation, follow your healthcare provider's treatment plan and dietary recommendations.

Remember that individual responses to lifestyle changes may vary, and it's essential to consult with a healthcare provider or registered dietitian for personalized advice and recommendations tailored to your specific needs and circumstances.

Seeking Medical Advice

Seeking medical advice is crucial when you experience health concerns or suspect that you may have a medical condition, including issues related to the gallbladder.

Here are steps to follow when seeking medical advice:

Recognize Symptoms: Pay attention to any symptoms you are experiencing.

Symptoms related to gallbladder issues can include abdominal pain, nausea, vomiting, and changes in stool color.

Consult a Primary Care Physician: Start by scheduling an appointment with your primary care physician (PCP) or general practitioner.

They can assess your symptoms, conduct a physical examination, and recommend initial tests if necessary.

Provide a Detailed Medical History: During your appointment, be prepared to provide a detailed medical history, including any pre-existing conditions, medications you're taking, and family history of gallbladder or digestive issues.

Describe Symptoms: Clearly describe your symptoms to your healthcare provider.

Mention the location, intensity, duration, and any factors that worsen or alleviate your symptoms.

Undergo Diagnostic Tests: Your healthcare provider may order diagnostic tests to evaluate your gallbladder and digestive system.

Common tests include ultrasound, blood tests, and sometimes a HIDA scan or an endoscopic procedure like an ERCP.

Consult a Specialist: If your PCP suspects gallbladder issues, they may refer you to a gastroenterologist or a surgeon for further evaluation and treatment.

Ask Questions: Don't hesitate to ask questions and seek clarification about your condition, treatment options, and any concerns you have.

Follow Medical Advice: Once you receive a diagnosis, it's essential to follow your healthcare provider's recommendations.

This may include dietary changes, medications, or surgical intervention, depending on the severity of your condition.

Maintain Communication: Keep an open line of communication with your healthcare provider.

Update them on any changes in your symptoms, medication side effects, or concerns.

Seek a Second Opinion (if necessary): If you are uncertain about your diagnosis or treatment plan, it's perfectly acceptable to seek a second opinion from another qualified healthcare provider.

Emergency Situations: If you experience severe abdominal pain, fever, jaundice (yellowing of the skin or eyes), or other concerning symptoms, seek immediate medical attention at the nearest emergency room. Remember that early detection and treatment of gallbladder issues can prevent complications and improve your overall quality of life.

Conclusion

In conclusion, prioritizing gallbladder health is essential for maintaining overall well-being and digestive comfort.

Whether you're proactively working to prevent gallbladder issues or managing an existing condition, your journey to gallbladder wellness involves a combination of informed choices, lifestyle adjustments, and medical guidance.

Understanding the symptoms of gallbladder problems, seeking timely medical evaluation, and following treatment recommendations are critical steps in this journey.

Dietary modifications, portion control, hydration, regular physical activity, and stress management play significant roles in supporting gallbladder health.

Remember that gallbladder health is a personal journey, and each individual's experience and needs may vary.

It's important to consult with healthcare professionals, such as primary care physicians, specialists, or registered dietitians, for personalized guidance and treatment plans tailored to your specific condition.

By taking proactive measures, making informed decisions, and embracing a healthier lifestyle, you can promote gallbladder wellness and enhance your overall quality of life.

Your dedication to gallbladder health is an investment in your long-term well-being and digestive comfort.

www.ingramcontent.com/pod-product-compliance
Lightning Source LLC
Chambersburg PA
CBHW050812260726

48660CB00004B/1377